Thought Moves

An inner guide to *active living.*

Wayne Phillips, Ph.D., FACSM, CIC®, CVS-FR

Cover image:
Lisa Elliot Design

Acknowledgments

I want to acknowledge the profound influence of Christina Marshall on my thinking in general, and on this book in particular.

Christina is Founder and CEO of Intrinsic Solutions International, which is both a company and a global movement. In a country where the word 'Visionary' is, more often than not, used merely as a synonym for 'unusual', Christina exemplifies the true sense of that word, best defined by the Center for Visionary Leadership www.visionarylead.org

> Visionary leaders are the builders of a new dawn, working with imagination, insight, and boldness. They present a challenge that calls forth the best in people and brings them together around a shared sense of purpose. They work with the power of intentionality and alignment with a higher purpose. Their eyes are on the horizon, not just on the near at hand. They are social innovators and change agents, seeing the big picture and thinking strategically.

I feel privileged to have received the benefit of her experience, mentoring and passion throughout my ongoing training as a Certified Intrinsic Coach® and a Certified Valuations Specialist. I look forward to continuing this connection in the future. This book is one of the outcomes of that connection. It is my (and only my) interpretation of my understanding of my thinking about.... my thinking.

Thank you Christina.

I also want to acknowledge my sister Denyse for her constant support in this project, and the many discussions we have had about 'thinking about thinking'. Although she is not a trained coach I know I can always rely on her laser keen perception and feedback. Nothing focuses the clarity of your writing more than when someone whose opinions you value says 'Ok, I read the piece you sent me... so what does it mean?'

Thanks Din.

When we need to make a difficult and important decision, we typically contrast one possible way of doing things with another. For example we say 'if I do this then this will happen, but if I do <u>this</u> then this (other thing) will happen!' Even if we make a 'pros and cons' list, it is often still hard to make a final decision based only on 'the arithmetic' since feelings often get in the way of counting, reason and logic ('It just doesn't feel right'). This can lead to frustrating circular conversations with ourselves which are complicated even further if we seek out the opinions and counsel of friends and family. With your best interests at heart they will tell you what they would do "If I was you" or "If I was in your place", two scenarios that are not only physically and psychologically impossible, but also not in <u>your own</u> best decision making interests! Only when you are able to clarify YOUR thinking about what is important TO YOU, will the best way forward be revealed FOR YOU. When this actually does happen it is almost always accompanied by an 'aha moment', sometimes with surprising results! This book provides an introduction to a powerful methodology that I call 'meta-thinking': It will provide a path towards clarifying **how you think about** important decisions in your life, vs simply **what you think about** them. The Best Thinking that emerges from this approach will enable you to more clearly set and achieve action-oriented goals.

Reading and reflecting on the **Thought Pieces** in the following pages can enable you to 'Think Differently' about what you value, and so elicit what is important to you in your unique, one of a kind, life.

When this occurs you will begin to experience the power of meta-thinking.

Thought Moves!

*You cannot solve a problem
from the same consciousness
that created it.
You must learn to see the world anew.*

~ Albert Einstein

Thinking Differently
– About this Book –

There are probably thousands of 'How To' books about starting to exercise or 'getting' more exercise, and when I use the word 'exercise' in this book, I mean physical activity in its broadest sense, from walking to working out.

Ok now I've got that out of the way, what's so different about this book?

Well, firstly, this is not a 'How to Do' book, It's not even a 'What to Do' book. In fact it does not focus at all on the 'Do' part: that will emerge all by itself, in a way that, hopefully, will become clear later.

I realize that this may initially seem a little strange: not at all like the usual way of things, not at all like the ways you have been used to thinking and reading and hearing about exercise.

Here are some other differences between this book and 99% of other books that claim to be able to 'get' you to exercise.
It contains

- No 'tips', 'guidance' or 'advice' for 'getting fit' and/or being more active
- Nothing about things like 'How to lose weight/reduce stress in 3 easy steps' (or any number of steps)
- Nothing about what you 'should' do or 'ought' to do
- Nothing about it being 'for your own good'
- No instructions in how to 'Pull yourself together/make a commitment/get serious' or (my favorite) 'Focus!'
- Nothing about 'Try harder' next time
- Nothing about how good you will feel 'If only you would do it'
- No mention of anything that sounds like 'Really ... it's not as hard as you think!'

All the things on this list represent what you could call a 'one up, one down' approach to change. This where I – as the (One Up) expert, bestow pearls of wisdom and instruction upon you, the (One Down) recipient. You will then (with grateful thanks) just get out there and do it! This all may sound very logical, or at least very familiar to you, if only because this is what happens out there most of the time. This is how the 'business' of exercise is conducted. However, history – and countless New Year's Resolution lists similar to the one above – has shown that this hardly ever works.

Another reason why this book contains no 'to do' lists, or 'have to do' lists like the one above, is that I'm pretty sure you have all read, heard, experienced, or said many of these kinds of things before. You already know this stuff and, as the saying goes … 'How's that working out for you?' The reality is that none of the 'dos' on these kinds of lists work for very long, if at all.

However, the most important reason why this book contains no lists is because any list I made up would be about things that **I** want you to do – or that **I** think you should do. In other words they would be **MY** things – they would be things about **ME** – about **MY** thinking about you. In contrast this book is about **YOU** – or rather it is about **your** thinking about **YOU**. If you want to get absolutely clear, what this book is really about is **your thinking about your thinking about YOU!**

I call this meta-thinking

It is something that most of us rarely do, or even think about doing. However, as I will lay out in the later sections of this book, it is something that can be of great value to us – once we become aware of the process! The **Thought Pieces** in this book are part of building this awareness. They were developed out of situations I was part of, or examples of circumstances that elicited a different kind of thinking from me. Some also developed out of conversations with fellow coaches. As I hope you will soon discover, 'thinking about thinking' is a powerful basis for clarity, and for valuing – two things that are the foundation of lasting change.

As you read – and reflect on – these **Pieces**, be open to and aware of any **Thoughts** that may come to your attention. Sometimes they will seem to come out of nowhere! Allow your **Thoughts** free rein – ponder what you have read and you may be surprised at what comes up for you!

I want this book to be as much a reflective process as a reading experience. So, after each **Thought Piece**, there is a "**Thoughts**" space, with an opportunity to reflect on and jot down what thoughts start to come up for you.

Reading and reflecting in this way can elicit new thinking – thinking that is drawn from the 'undermind', that place we all have that exists just below the level of consciousness. This kind of thinking is constant and ongoing and can be brought to awareness only by allowing time for slower reflection – by thinking about your thinking. This is where the foundations of our values are formed and is the basis of the choices you make in your own one-of-a-kind life. It is where true clarity lives.

When this moment of clarity – this 'aha moment' – hits, you will truly start to feel that **Thought Moves** – to wherever you want to be, to wherever you want to go, to whatever is important to you. Of singular importance is that these thoughts will be inspired by your own unique values and experiences, rather than, as is so often the case, by other people's opinions, advice or 'guidance'.

The approach I introduce in this book is based in part on my academic background: in my training and experience as a wellness-oriented behavioral scientist. In the main however it is centered around my extensive training and experience as an Intrinsic Coach® and a Certified Valuations Specialist, using the Marshall-Hartman Synthesis of the Hartman Value Profile as a coaching tool. While the major focus of this book is on exercise and/or being more active, the value principles on which it is based are universal and can be applied to any goal.

> *Thought Moves us in an infinite number of ways.*
> *Noticing those thoughts and becoming aware of the value*
> *of those thoughts clarifies the ways.*

Thought Pieces

If only they would 3
The F Word 7
Nothing Happens until Something Moves 10
Be a High(er) Energy User, Not a Low(er) Energy User ... 13
JAMM (Just A Mite More) 16
Kicking Yourself Up the Assets 20
Getting Less Bad 23
GOOOAAAALLLLL!!!!!! 26
Think Different – Do Different – Be Different 29
Little by Little 32
Options, Actions, Directions 35
Windmills of the Mind 39
With a Little Help from Your Friends 43
Asking the Expert – Making Your Own Difference 46

Thinking INSIDE the Box
Get S.M.A.R.T.! (Look Yourself in the i) 51
Thinking iS.M.A.R.T., Specifically 54
Thinking iS.M.A.R.T., Measurably 57
Thinking iS.M.A.R.T., Attainably 60
Thinking iS.M.A.R.T., Relevantly (Really Importantly) .. 63
Thinking iS.M.A.R.T., Timely 65
Thinking iS.M.A.R.T.A., Accountably 67

Thinking About Choices – A Workshop 69

Next Steps: The Thinking Behind Choices 75
The Hartman/Marshall Synthesis 76

A Special Offer for YOU! 79

If only they would...

I grew up in the UK as a jock, (though we don't call it that over there). I was captain of teams and loved to work out – two things central to my life back then. I even used to skip classes on occasion to get an extra work out and (gladly) suffered the consequences if caught. I finally buckled down, went through college as a Physical Education (PE) teacher, taught PE in High School (though we don't call it that over there) and later became Physical Education Director at London Central YMCA in London, England. This was where my own real-life learning began, and, all unknowing, I first started to become aware of the power and value of **Thought Moves**.

I was still heavily into sports and fitness at this time – and still socialized with others of the same ilk. My new job at the Y however was another thing entirely! As PE Director I had to deal more and more with people who (I perceived) were not at all like me. It was bad enough that they did not exercise but – horror of horrors – they didn't even <u>like</u> to exercise! I remember being frustrated with these people because they clearly knew (and would tell me repeatedly) that they 'should' exercise. In fact it often seemed to me that their only reason for doing exercise was because they knew that they 'should' do it – that they 'ought' to do it – and – it almost goes without saying of course that most of them had also been 'meaning to' do it for some time. What was wrong with these people? If only they would be more active – they would feel great!

Part of my job was to promote the Y programs and 'get' people to participate. Every month at new member's orientation I would stand up and extol the virtues of the Y and the even greater ones of exercise. I would be amusing, motivating and informative (Ok I'm just saying that's what people told me!). Because of this – at least on the surface, and particularly on that evening – things always appeared to bode well for the future activity levels of our members. The reality, however, was something (as Monty Python would say) Completely Different!

I couldn't believe how silly these people were (I used different adverbs and adjectives back in those days). How did these intelligent, concerned, and initially 'motivated' members end up by giving up and not following my directions! After all I was the expert – that's why they came to me – and <u>they came to me</u> remember! However, what usually happened was after a few days, a few weeks, or sometimes a few months, most of them had stopped working out.

Oh, they would still come to the Y – maybe for a sauna, the coffee shop, the tanning beds or a friendly game of doubles badminton – the latter typically involving laughter but little foot movement!! Some of them were also avoiding me! What was wrong with these people? If only they would be more active – they would see I was right!

I couldn't believe how they did not appreciate – or could not be motivated by – the amazing benefits they could get from exercise – from working out regularly. This prompted many 'what's wrong with these people' conversations with my fellow Y workers (all of them jocks and/or ex PE teachers).

Now don't get me wrong – I did not give these people highly intensive workouts – I was an 'expert' with a deal of common sense! I would spend a lot of time with them, talk to them about how good they would feel – caution them to start off slowly and carefully, and gradually work up the intensity. By the way, this remains the default approach even today – traditional attitudes still dominate!).

As my years at the Y progressed I began to realize that (to my amazement), most people <u>really</u> did not like to work out – and it was my friends and I who were the minority. It was we, in fact, who were the oddballs, and ironically as I later discovered, many of those inactive Y members I worked with were also saying about us 'They work out all the time – What's wrong with these people?' What an eye opener that was!

My response was to begin to focus even more on trying to make working out as 'user friendly' as possible – telling people to start with easier and lower intensity approaches, stressing the importance of slow progression and re-iterating the benefits of getting fit. I did get some improvement in adherence but really not that much more. What's wrong with these people? If only they would be more active – they would see and feel the benefits!

In retrospect I now look back at this time and realize I was really just giving them the same old routines – the same old story. I got much better at telling that story, explaining things in advance and clarifying issues, though always from my own perspective. There was not much ***Thought*** in my own **Moves** at that stage of my life. I got better at dealing with people (so I thought) at relating to people (so I thought) and at empathizing with people (so I thought). Still, it wasn't enough – still they didn't continue – what the heck was going on here? What was wrong with these people? If only they would...

Skip forward a few decades and I am now Professor Emeritus at Arizona State University (ASU) and the Keynote Speaker at a major Aging Conference. My topic was related to 'Healthy Aging', and the audience consisted of well over two hundred physicians, nurses, and case managers, all of whom were dedicated to healthy, active aging. As part of my approach I talked about the importance of being active throughout life and how ineffective current approaches and guidelines had been to 'get' older adults to be active. As a sort of 'litmus test' for this I asked the audience a single question

Question: *How many of you think that 'exercising', or simply being regularly active is 'good for you' from a health and medicine perspective?*
Response: Everyone raised their hand.

I then said: *The Centers for Disease Control define 'regularly active' as participating in physical activity/exercise for at least 4 days per week at a level at least as hard as a brisk walk and continuing this for at least 6 months. Those of you who have followed this guideline please keep your hands raised and those who haven't please lower your hands.*
Response: Only about 1/3 of the audience kept their hands raised (roughly in line with national statistics)

So there I was getting a similar kind of reaction from some of the most knowledgeable individuals in the Arizona health care world: the same reaction I got all those years ago at the Y. What's going on here? (What's wrong with these people? If only they would...)

Increasingly the answer to this repeating (and rather judgmental) question had started appearing to be much broader and less simplistic than I had initially assumed. Either this audience, together with approximately 70% of the country, were just plain lazy and/or stupid (My YMCA thinking), or <u>it's something else</u>.

It was this realization – one that gradually dawned on me sometime between the UK and the US, somewhere between the YMCA and ASU – that gave me my first real sense of the power of **Thought Moves**.

It's all about the something else!

thoughts

The F Word

FUN! I was thinking about that word the other day. I was reading something that said when people want to be more active they should 'make it fun' or 'find something that is fun' or even 'find something you enjoy'. I see these same kind of suggestions in some of the annually recycled 'ten sure-fire tips' to stick to your New Year Resolution's exercise program (Déjà vu all over again?). Of course if you can find an exercise that <u>is</u> Fun, and remains Fun, then you are likely on your way to a long-term love affair with exercise and your active lifestyle is virtually assured. My point here however is that if you look only for Fun or if you think it always has to be Fun, your options are more likely to be limited, and your intentions are more likely to be compromised.

What prompted this line of thinking was a conversation I had while standing next to a lady doing some walking on a treadmill (She was doing the walking, I was doing the standing). We were chatting about the usual kind of stuff 'How do I get rid of my flabby arms?', 'What's the best kind of exercise to lose weight?', etc. I was talking about the fact that she was already doing something really positive by walking on a regular basis when she said 'But this isn't fun'. To which my response was 'Who said it had to be fun?'

Of course this got a big laugh from her and her neighboring treadmill walker who automatically thought that the 'jock' in me was speaking. However that was not the point I was trying to make. The day before, this lady had seen me in the gym as I was coming to the end of a fairly intense session on the elliptical trainer. There I was in front of her, cranking away, sweat flying, arms pumping. I asked her 'When you saw me on the elliptical yesterday, did it look like I was having Fun?' Again she and her neighbors laughed but (without quoting the resulting conversation word for word), the point I tried to make in the ensuing conversation was that, while I was definitely experiencing a number of positive physical and mental feelings during my workout, 'Fun' was not an appropriate descriptor of what these feelings were. Empowerment, self esteem, a sense of achievement, ego, being in control of my body, a sense of completion, of being in tune with the rhythm of my movements – any of those – or more – could describe what I was feeling. But FUN? This didn't even come close.

FUN is defined in the dictionary as 'enjoyment or playfulness', or 'something that provides mirth or amusement'. It is certainly a pleasant feeling, and one that almost by definition, is transient. In other words, it is not something likely to persuade you to adopt any kind of long-term behavior change (like regular exercise).

I said to this lady 'I see you here on a regular basis, so what is important to you about being here?' She thought for a while (actually for about 20 steps at 4 mph), and said. 'It's walking with my friend here (pointing to the lady on the next treadmill). We chat about things and the time just goes by'. In response to this I also let some time go by. Then she said, 'You know what the best thing is? When we walk out of the door at the end of the session, I feel really good about myself because I have achieved something'.

Sounds to me like a lot more than 'Fun'!

So as you think about this story –
what is important to you about being active?

thoughts

Nothing Happens until Something Moves

I was listening recently to Dr. Wayne Dyer's audio book of the Tao Te Ching (*Change your thoughts, change your life*). Verse 59 was about 'Living untroubled by good or bad fortune' and in his analysis of this verse Dr. Dyer mentioned the Albert Einstein quote, which is the title of this thought piece 'Nothing happens until something moves'. As I meditated after this verse it came to me that although Einstein was talking mainly through the medium of physics, this quote also applies to lifestyle change – and to meaningful goal achievement. So here's my Tao-inspired thinking about this

Meaningful lifestyle change is all about setting 'action oriented goals' – which involves two sets of 'movements':

the thinking, and the action

While it is true that 'nothing happens until something moves', it is also true that nothing happens until someone thinks, and so (stay with me here Albert!) no <u>different</u> movement (or behavior) can result without <u>different</u> thinking. Ok, take a deep breath and read that again slowly, I know I'm going to!

The point I am making here is that the first 'movement' has to be one that starts inside your head – a '**Thought Move**' away from your usual thinking – an 'aha' moment, however small. I talk about this in more detail in the last section of the book, but, briefly, without this first 'different thinking' there will be no different movement. Even though 'something may move' physically, there will be no lasting change.

Nothing different happens without different thinking.
Usual continues Usual, Different produces Different.

This is the embodiment of all our **Thought Moves**.
So … two questions:

1. If you are doing 'the usual' what does 'the different' look like to you?
2. What **Thought** is happening to **Move** you?

Think (differently) about it – make a **Thought Move**

thoughts

Be a High(er) Energy User, Not a Low(er) Energy User

Opened up my email one morning and found a reference to something called 'Parkour' and 'Free Running'. Since both of these were described as related to being active outdoors I checked them out. Parkour was initially developed in France and the name was taken from *parcours du combattant*, the classic obstacle course method of military training proposed by Georges Hébert a pioneering French physical educator, theorist and instructor. Free Running was developed out of Parkour. Here's the official definition of Parkour, in part...

> *Parkour is the art of moving through your environment using only your body and the surroundings to propel yourself. It can include running, jumping, climbing, even crawling, if that is the most suitable movement for the situation... it is better to consider Parkour as defined by the intention instead of the movements themselves. If the intention is to get somewhere using the most effective movements with the least loss of momentum, then it could probably be considered Parkour.*

Although it is not described as an 'extreme sport' the movements in all of the videos I looked at would be pretty 'hairy' for most individuals, and at least from my first brief look, suitable only for highly active people in great shape – or willing to train up to great shape. My 16 year old son has latched on to this experience and is now a Parkour runner 'par excellence'! *O Tempora, O Mores!*

Which brings me to my title above which is based on a quote taken from Per-Olaf Astrand, regarded as the grandfather of Exercise Physiology. The original quote was 'Be a high energy user, not a low energy user'. He was of the opinion, way back in the 1960s, that people could get great health benefits from using just a little more energy throughout the day. I address this issue more in "JAMM" below. While Parkour certainly does this, and much, much more, most of us can gain our health benefits at far lower and more manageable levels of exertion!

So, although in the US as a nation, we are seeking to lower energy costs and energy usage we, as individuals, will be far better off by taking the opposite path! Expend your own personal energy with abandon! Take a regular everyday activity (e.g. vacuuming) and do it a little faster. A word of caution however, although the Robin Williams vacuuming scene in 'Mrs. Doubtfire' certainly utilizes the 'higher energy user' principle, in my expert opinion this is a little extreme! More like 'Free Vacuuming'!

Most tasks in life can be done at a slightly elevated speed over a slightly longer time, or with just a little more effort (see below). Research has shown that anyone can get great health benefits by adopting this 'higher energy user' approach to life. Go a little faster, go a little longer.

So ... as you think about this and the tasks in your life
... what's coming up for you?

thoughts

JAMM
(Just A Mite More)

To follow up on my 'be a higher energy user' thought piece above, I wanted to talk a little about the Surgeon General's Report (SGR) on Physical Activity and Health (and you thought The SGR was all about smoking!). The brightest and best scientists in wellness, exercise and epidemiology compiled the SGR. It was released way back in 1996 and was an enormous and exhaustive review of the scientific literature that examined the effect of physical activity on health. Their findings still resonate today. The 'Physical Activity' in the title was defined as

> '... any bodily movement produced by skeletal muscles
> that results in energy expenditure'.

Ok, I know, I know, scientists tend to use lots of words, but really all they were saying here is that almost any kind of movement would count as physical activity. Their summary of all this research (the SGR was almost an inch thick) was contained in a single sentence.

> 'Every American should accumulate 30 minutes or more of moderate
> intensity physical activity on most, preferably all days of the week'

'Moderate intensity' was any activity that felt about as hard as a brisk walk. So what this means is that if you do something that feels about as hard as a brisk walk and do it in short bouts throughout the day that added up to around 30 minutes, you would get <u>great</u> health benefits! How cool is that!

You would also start feeling better, looking better, doing better. The <u>really</u> cool thing is that the 'something' you do that feels as hard as a brisk walk, doesn't have to be the same 'something' every time! So, 10 minutes of vacuuming (at a faster pace than usual) in the morning, 10 minutes of brisk walking before lunch and 10 minutes of raking leaves (at a faster pace than usual), would give you 30 minutes of 'moderate intensity physical activity'. Here's a hint: Make everything 'Just **A Mite More**'. We will see more **JAMM** examples later.

This almost sounds too good to be true! However, more than 5 decades of peer-reviewed research supports this approach. Take my word for it.

So all those years ago – with technology and exercise physiology still in its infancy – Per-Olaf Astrand's recommendation to 'Be a high energy user, not a low energy user', really nailed it! What a guy!

The final thing to say on this subject is that these same SGR scientists also calculated that 30 minutes of 'moderate intensity physical activity' worked out to around **150 Calories**. You could expend this number of calories by doing some things for a shorter time at a higher intensity and some things for a longer time at a lower intensity – and still receive the same health benefits! Here's a sample list – but you get the idea – right?

- Washing and waxing a car – 45-60 minutes
- Washing windows or floors – 45-60 minutes
- Playing volleyball – 45 minutes
- Playing touch football – 30-45 minutes
- Gardening – 30-45 minutes
- Wheeling self in wheelchair – 30-40 minutes
- Walking 1¼ miles in 35 minutes (20 min/mile)
- Basketball (shooting baskets) – 30 minutes
- Bicycling 5 miles – 30 minutes
- Dancing fast (social) – 30 minutes
- Pushing a stroller 1½ miles in 30 minutes
- Raking leaves – 30 minutes
- Walking 2 miles in 30 minutes (15 min/mile)
- Water aerobics – 30 minutes
- Swimming laps – 20 minutes
- Wheelchair basketball – 20 minutes
- Basketball (playing a game) – 15-20 minutes
- Bicycling 4 miles in 15 minutes
- Jumping rope – 15 minutes
- Running 1½ miles in 15 minutes (10 min/mile)
- Shoveling snow – 15 minutes
- Stair walking – 15 minutes

Lower Intensity
More Time

Higher Intensity
Less Time

NOTE: Adapted from SGR guidelines 1996

With some thought and intention, your chores, as well as many of the things you do – or have to do – on a regular basis (Known as activities of daily living – ADL) can be used to move you to become a 'higher energy user'

How do you know how much energy you are using? Well the intuitive way is to do something you usually do but 'just a mite more'. The second and more quantitative way is to look at how each activity has been officially measured for its energy expenditure. *The Compendium of Physical Activities* is a scientific publication that pulls together a list of hundreds of different ADL with their energy costs. You can easily find this with an online search.

Some of these ADL options above may work for you and some may not. There are also many more options, limited only by your own imagination! So, as you think about this information and your lifestyle, in your own home and in your own environment …

… *what's JAMMing for you?*

thoughts

Kicking Yourself Up the Assets

Taking an asset-based, or positive approach to life is often viewed as a 'glass half empty, glass half full' situation. But I think it is much more than that. The growing field of Positive Psychology has demonstrated, time and again, that viewing things from an asset-based, positive or optimistic manner is far more than just 'Positive Thinking' which I think for most people has more of the feel of the philosophy espoused by Stuart Smalley, late of *Saturday Night Live*, who, while looking at himself in the mirror, affirms 'I'm good enough, I'm smart enough, and doggone it, people like me!'

Educational research out of Stanford University in the 1980's with teachers and teaching performance, reported that an approach focusing and building on the teacher's '<u>assets</u>' (i.e. their strengths, and what they were doing well) promoted high quality learning, while an approach focusing on the teacher's '<u>deficits</u>' (i.e. their weaknesses, and correcting what they were doing 'wrong') was far less effective in eliciting quality learning. Yet this 'deficit-based' approach is still out there in education, in exercise, and in behavior change.

As an example of this, one of the best known hypotheses in the area of Successful Aging is 'The Compression of Morbidity'. This refers to the idea that the period of decline and sickness (Morbidity) typically experienced at the end of life may be reduced (Compressed) by adopting healthier lifestyles. This hypothesis has received much attention in the field of gerontology and as a professor I have talked about it myself on many occasions.

With my **Thought Moves** hat on however, I see that, although this hypothesis was clearly aimed at doing good, it was actually taking a 'getting less bad' approach (See my next **Thought Piece**). Not much asset-kicking going on here! Instead there is an obvious dichotomy between 'Successful Aging', which is a positive, asset-based concept, and 'The Compression of Morbidity' which is a negative, deficit-based concept.

So here's my **Thought Moves**, asset-kicking version of this hypothesis. You read it here first!

Instead of 'Compression' – why not 'Expansion'?
Instead of 'Morbidity' – why not 'Mobility'?

And so we have 'The Expansion of Mobility'. In other words 'being better, longer' instead of 'being worse, shorter'. I know which one I would choose!

So as you think about situations
and what is important in your life –
what assets are kicking up for you?

thoughts

Getting Less Bad

When I was a professor at Arizona State University, I was invited to be lead author on a book chapter in a major work called *The Handbook of Health Psychology*. The title of the chapter was 'Effects of physical activity on physical and psychological health: Implications for exercise adherence and psychophysiological mechanisms'. A pretty long and involved title I admit, but then this was a pretty long and involved book: I was actually Chapter 38 out of 51! The reason I bring this up here is that it was in my research for writing that chapter I was first struck by the fact that almost everything on 'psychological health' out there in the scientific literature at the time was about 'getting less bad'.

I still see the same thing out there today. The rationale for wellness goals such as getting active, getting fit, or eating healthy are predominantly based either on reducing your <u>actual</u> 'bad stuff' or on reducing your <u>risk</u> of 'bad stuff'. With a moment's thought you could probably come up with your own list of the usual 'bad stuff' we are told we have to get less of: inactivity, overweight, obesity, high blood pressure, high blood sugar, high stress, depression, anxiety, risk of a heart attack, risk of a stroke, risk of dying, etc.

I suspect this is a consequence of living with our current Medical Model of health, which is uniquely designed to kick in and fix the 'bad stuff', and has little or no designs at all on the 'good stuff'. The result of this is that we tend to view our wellbeing more in terms of how bad we aren't rather than how good we are.

In a similar way, when we try to set and achieve wellness goals we are typically taught to focus almost as much on overcoming obstacles to these goals rather than achieving the goal itself; to focus on what we are <u>not</u> 'getting' rather on what we <u>are</u> 'getting'. It reminds me of the lady I described in **The F Word** (page 7). Even though she was truly gaining – and feeling – significant and meaningful benefits from her regular walking, her first response was to focus on what she wasn't getting 'It's not fun'.

What I know as an Intrinsic Coach®, Certified Valuations Specialist and behavioral scientist, is that focusing on the positive aspects of pursuing an active lifestyle will bring you a host of positive benefits. You will look better and feel better about your self and your life, be more alert, have more energy, clearer thinking, have a better quality of life, better sleep. But Wait! There's more …

The old clichéd distinction between people who either view 'the glass half empty or the glass half full' reveals a pathway to some major (and positive!) consequences. Research has shown that people who have a more optimistic (i.e. positive, glass half full) view of things do better in life: they earn more money, are more successful, have more friends and even live longer. As if this wasn't positive enough, you can even <u>learn</u> to be positive! You think I'm joking? Go check out the research and writings of Dr. Martin Seligman, acknowledged as the founder of 'Positive Psychology'. He has written three best-selling books on the power of positive thinking (*Learned Optimism*, *Authentic Happiness*, and *Flourish*). Another leading Positive Psychology advocate, Shawn Achor, has also described how we can learn to be positive, in his two books, *The Happiness Advantage* and *Before Happiness*. Reading any of these will put a lot of things into (a more positive) perspective.

So … As you read about these benefits –
what positive thoughts and feelings are coming up for you?

thoughts

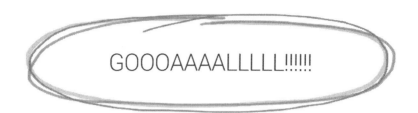

GOOOAAAALLLLLL!!!!!!

Achieving a wellness goal can often be as exciting as scoring a soccer goal – maybe not quite as vocal as that famous Spanish Soccer commentator's signature screeeeeeeeeem of joy – but still something that feels pretty good!

And here's the thing – even if you don't achieve the goal you have set for yourself (NOOOOO!) your 'failure' can still be viewed as something positive (YEEEEESSSSSS!). It all depends on how you choose to think about it – on how your **Thought Moves** you.

William James, a 19th Century philosopher who also wrote influential books on the, then emerging, science of psychology, wrote

The greatest weapon against stress
is our ability to choose one thought over another.

… and he emphasized that we all can learn to make that choice.

This thinking can also apply to the stress we feel when 'failing' to make our goal, something I learned during my 4 decades in the field of Wellness. My training as an Intrinsic Coach® and Certified Valuation Specialist brought even more clarity to this. There is a very effective and usable process for the setting of action oriented goals (more later). However, what is important to you, and unique to you, is how you <u>choose to react</u> to either achieving or not achieving those goals. It is this, more than anything, that will determine how you continue – or whether you continue – to progress.

The choice of thinking here is between 'Failure' or 'Learning'. In choosing Learning ('I didn't make my goal – What did I learn from this?'), you are far more likely to ultimately achieve your Goal than choosing Failure ('I didn't make my goal – Why the #$%@ did I screw up?'). See also **Windmills of the Mind** (page 39).

The really cool thing about this approach is that 'What did I Learn?' is equally powerful <u>whatever happens with your goal</u>.

You did it? What did you learn? What's next?

You didn't do it? What did you learn? What's next?

So as you think about goals you have set –
what did you learn – what's coming up for you?

thoughts

Think Different – Do Different – Be Different

We have known for several decades now that simply providing people with accurate, easy to understand information about exercise and wellness is no guarantee that they will ultimately act on this information. Never before, on the web and in the media, have we had such a wealth of easily accessible information about paths to active, healthy living and, simultaneously, never before have we had such a prevalence of inactivity and obesity/overweight in the US.

Clearly knowledge and education are not sufficient agents for change. Yet most of the approaches in wellness and exercise continue to provide the same information over and over again and continue to expect it to work (this time).

Hold on a second ... That reminds me of something

> *Insanity: doing the same thing over and over again*
> *and expecting a different result*
> ~ Albert Einstein

Hmmm ...time for a different way of thinking – Time for a ***Thought Move***.

I have posted some 'thinking' options below which could perhaps be the start of a different direction for some of you reading this book. It is not an exhaustive list by any means but hopefully can serve as starting point 'options'. Options are possibilities drawn from **Thought Moves** that contain a range of actions and choices that could bridge the gap between what you want and what you achieve.

These are not meant to be guidelines or instructions. Some of the 'options' have been part of my thinking for a while, and some came to me as I was thinking about and writing this **Thought Piece**. They all have an evidence-based background.

Different thinking vs usual thinking

- **Different:** Adopt a positive attitude and approach to exercise and physical activity and emphasize achieving your goal.
- **Usual:** Once you have set your goal, think of all the obstacles that can get in your way and then think of ways to avoid or overcome those obstacles (HUH?).

Research has shown that an 'asset-based' (goal oriented) approach is consistently more effective than a 'deficit-based" (obstacle overcoming) approach

- **Different:** Focus on getting 'more good' i.e. the positive benefits of exercise and activity (more energy, more alertness, greater self-confidence).
- **Usual:** focus on getting 'less bad' (reduce high blood pressure, reduce anxiety, stress etc.).

Was it Frank Sinatra that sang "Ac-centuate the Positive … E-liminate the Negative"? That gentleman was ahead of his (wellness) time!

- **Different:** The expert provides opportunities <u>for clients</u> to think about and clarify what is important <u>to them</u> about exercise.
- **Usual:** Expert stresses what is 'good for' the client about exercise, and then tells them how to do it

NOTE: this is <u>not</u> the same thing – think about it!

- **Different:** Consistently provide stories and examples illustrating that heath and regular exercise is easier to achieve than most people realize. It's never been as easy as this to get active!
- **Usual:** Typically 'just do it' or 'I just have to do it' or 'I should do it' or even 'no pain no gain'.

- **Different:** Consistently 'reframe' exercise and physical activity (with lots of examples, case studies and research) so it is presented and viewed as an integral part of a normal, enjoyable life.
- **Usual:** Exercise is necessary and something that just has to be endured. Something that interferes with your life – or has to be done in addition to everything else you have to do. What a drag!

What options are coming up for you?

Think about it …

thoughts

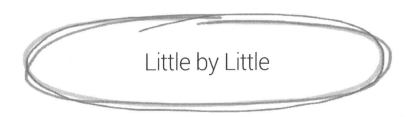

Little by Little

When I was in my earliest years as a university professor I remember my proud mother asking what exactly it was that I did as 'Dr. Phillips'. I said something like "I do a lot of research to find out what the benefits of exercise are for older people". She replied, "Why do you need to do that? Everybody knows that exercise is good for you – especially if you are older". My whole carefully planned research agenda crushed by a loving parent in two short sentences!

Like my mother you've probably also heard that exercise is 'good for you' and you've probably heard it most of your life. It's one of those conventional wisdoms that everybody knows is true and has always been true. As a scientist I can tell you that, although exercise is certainly an important path to good health and wellness, contrary to conventional wisdom, 'exercise' (and especially the 'getting fit' way most people think about it), is not the only path. There is now overwhelming evidence that just being more active 'little by little' throughout the day can elicit meaningful health benefits. Although this is clearly good news for all adults – it is not exactly new news.

Way back in 1961 two physicians, Hans Kraus and Wilhelm Raab published a book entitled 'Hypokinetic Disease: diseases produced by lack of exercise'. More than 50 years ago these two physicians were warning against the dangers of inactivity. Here's a quote from their opening chapter:

> "When we analyze our daily lives, we can see how the active function of our muscles has been taken over step by step by labor saving devices. We do not walk, but ride; we do not climb stairs, but use elevators; we do not lift anything of any weight, but we have devices that do that lifting for us. Most of the chores that used to require a certain amount of physical activity have been taken over by machines. We do not mow our lawns by pushing a lawnmower – it is become motorized. We have push

> *button heating, we have vacuum cleaners, and we have
> dishwashers. In short we do not move at all."*

Here's another early quote that really grabbed me:

> *"From the crib to the playpen, to the television set,
> perambulator and school bus, our children are raised as a
> sedentary race, domesticated even from the first day of
> their lives"*

Wow! This is really telling it like it is! However, more than 50 years later
we are still telling the same story.

More positively slanted evidence came some 35 years after Kraus and
Raab, with The Surgeon General's Report on Physical Activity and
Health. Published in 1996, this was a massive review of the health and
exercise literature. It examined and analyzed literally thousands of studies
on the health benefits of endurance/aerobic activities of various kinds.
While they did confirm the existing belief that 'fitness' or 'vigorous
exercise' was beneficial to health, there was a very surprising 'kicker' to this
news. They discovered that physical activity of what they called 'moderate
intensity' could provide major health benefits for previously sedentary
or insufficiently active individuals. This is the summary sentence of their
Report that I used to make all my undergraduates memorize (!)

> *Every American should accumulate 30 minutes or more of
> moderate intensity physical activity on most, preferably all,
> days of the week.*

I have written about this in more detail earlier (See **JAMM**, page 16)
but, briefly, what they called 'moderate intensity physical activity' could
be <u>any activity that felt about as hard as a brisk walk.</u> This could include
everyday activities such as household chores, mowing the lawn or raking
leaves. If you look for new ways to include these types of activities at this
level every day, it will increase your stamina (aerobic fitness) and significantly
improve the way you feel. In other words you can, little by little, adopt
a more active and healthier lifestyle. All you have to do is 'Just a Mite
More'. That's it! Great news for everyone who doesn't like to exercise!

Not that my mother would have been too impressed with me telling her
what she already knew!

> **So – as you think about moderate intensity activity –
> what is coming up for you, little by little?**

thoughts

Options, Actions, Directions

If history is any judge, telling people what to do is not a great way to elicit behavior change. As I have commented many times in different ways in different **Thought Pieces**, goals are best achieved when they are truly/intrinsically important to the individual involved and when they have 'ownership' of the goal, and the actions and directions leading to its achievement.

However, offering 'options' rather than 'instructions' or 'tips' can be one way of eliciting this kind of 'intrinsic thinking'. Options are possibilities that contain a range of actions and choices that could bridge the gap between what an individual wants and their achievement of that 'want'. Options are potentials, whether looking at choices, actions, resources, perspectives or opinions.

So ... here are some options that have worked for many people who were ready to become more active. Some of these may work for you and some may not. Some may not even be possible for you or desirable to you – but may prompt a **Thought** that **Moves** you in a direction – one that you value, but just hadn't thought about until now.

- The 'doc' Option: Actually, this first one is a recommendation! Although for the great majority of people, exercise is both safe and beneficial, I recommend that you first talk to your doctor about your ideas and options for becoming active before you start any kind of activity program. Include him or her in your options – they will definitely be interested! The American Medical Association and the American College of Sports Medicine are collaborators on an initiative called 'Exercise is Medicine'. This recommends that physicians become more knowledgeable about, and involved in, the physical activity goals of their patients. If you have questions about being active that your doctor can't answer – or even if he/she can answer – ask to be referred to a qualified wellness educator or trainer. You can also refer your physician to the 'Exercise is Medicine' website – they'll thank you for it! Google it now!

- The 'family and friends' Option: Research has shown that one option for activity is social support. In other words people are more likely to start and continue to be active if they have the support of others. So, for example, you could ask a family member, or a friend, to join you on your regular walks. This then becomes more of a social event than 'exercise' or 'a workout'. Perhaps you can find someone who enjoys – or would like to enjoy – spending some active time with you – from grandchildren to grandparents and everyone in between. Think about and talk to your family about 'energy using' ideas around the house or outside the house and incorporate them into your active lifestyle plan. Make it a game for you and/or your children.

- The 'Just A Mite More' Option: Shopping, doing errands and even housework or chores can also be a way to add activity into your life. I talked about this in earlier **Thought Pieces,** but it always bears repeating. The great thing here is that to elicit any benefits, this 'exercise that isn't really exercise' option only has to be at moderate intensity. Once you have internalized the principles from this information, then you have endless options to **Be a Higher Energy User, Not a Lower Energy User** (page 13).

- The 'extra steps' Option: A simple and inexpensive 'activity monitor' (like Fitbit e.g.), can keep count of your daily activity in terms of the number of steps you take each day. However, here's something to make a note of. When you purchase or even read about these devices, you will no doubt discover that you 'need' to do 10,000 steps per day to receive any health benefits. This is really over-simplifying things, so don't get discouraged by this enormous number – physical activity is not solely about arithmetic. Look back at our 3rd option above and simply do 'Just a Mite More'. In other words use your device to track how many steps you usually take in a day (record 2 or 3 days and take the average) and then look for ways to add more steps to this total. Progress one step at a time! FYI, 'activity monitors' are now known as 'wearable monitors' (or 'wearables'). They are designed almost like fashion accessories and can, for example, be worn on the wrist. They are smaller and more sophisticated and, in addition to steps, can track distance, sleep, energy expenditure, diet, and hydration levels. You can even synch these devices to your computer and smart phone (yes there is an app for that!). Using these devices you are also able to work with a coach who can pull up your data remotely on a web-based 'dashboard' and use it as a coaching tool. This exciting and cutting edge technology has great potential to enable people to move toward a more active lifestyle. If you are curious to know more, please contact me and I will be happy to provide some reliable resources.

- The 'get stronger' Option: I have left the best until last here (my opinion!). Strength training has developed a bad 'rep' over the years – especially for older adults. Myths abound about how it is 'too dangerous at my age', or 'it's only for men – younger men'. However, more than a decade of scientific research has shown that individuals of any age can benefit from strength training. An overwhelming amount of research has reported positive changes in both cardiovascular and musculoskeletal health with strength training – particularly the high intensity type. Be sure to choose a well-qualified coach or trainer. Do your homework and you will reap the benefits!

So, as you think about these options above …
What's coming up that is important to you?

thoughts

Windmills of the Mind

As we think about what we 'should' do in our quest for health and wellness (and, too often, why we don't do it!) we frequently find our thoughts blowing around and around inside our head just like one of those child's hand held colored windmills. As I was writing this, it reminded me of the words of that Michel Legrand song of the late 60's, 'Windmills of your Mind'

> *'Like a circle in a spiral, like a wheel within a wheel,*
> *never ending or beginning, on an ever-spinning reel ... '*

That's what those 'should' thoughts mostly feel like – "I know I should do this because ... but I know I usually don't do it ... but if I don't do it, then what? ... What if I do it ... I wish I would do it ... but when I start I never finish... and if ...? and if ...? etc, etc?" Or those negative 'Why' thoughts – "why do I always do this? ... why can't I succeed? ... why do I never stick to something? ... why do I always fail?"

I'm sure we've all had those kinds of thoughts before –

> *'round and round and round they go and where they stop nobody knows!'*

Let's use exercise as an example. You want to become more active and you have achieved this for a few days or even a few weeks ... but then you just stop. What's the problem here? You know that you <u>should</u> exercise and you know <u>why</u> you should do it – but you just stop. You have done this before and each time you 'fail', you go round and around in your head wondering why you always do this, and ultimately decide that maybe you just didn't try hard enough.

What is going on here? Does this happen to everyone all the time? Are we all just lazy (because we just can't be bothered to do it) or stupid (because we know what is 'good for us' but don't do it anyway?).

Of course not!

It is something much more basic than this. Very often it is the <u>kind</u> of question you ask (yourself or others) that 'pre-selects' not only the way you set your goal, but also the way you set your mind. At the same time this kind of question sets your response to making (or, especially, not making) the goal, as well as your <u>next</u> attempt at the goal. Here's my **Thought Moves** take on this, based on current coaching research and behavioral science.

'Why?' questions are almost always the first ones to be asked after the fact. If you set yourself a goal and you don't make that goal, I can almost guarantee the first thing your trainer will ask (or you will ask yourself) is some variation of 'Why?' – "Why do you think you didn't make that goal?" This is hardly ever productive: if asked of another person, they tend to produce defensive answers ("I just got too busy", "I just didn't feel like it" etc.). If asked of yourself, they tend to produce some variation of "I don't know", followed by "Maybe I could do this, or maybe I could have done that, or next time maybe, maybe, maybe …"

… never ending or beginning like an ever spinning reel!

More productive and far less circular are 'What?' questions. Not a "What should I do?" kind of question, since that's really the same thing we just talked about above. A different and more clarifying question is "<u>What is important</u> to me (about this goal)?" It is essential to say here that this is not the same as "What is best for me?", or 'What is good for me', or "What will benefit me?", or even "What will I get out of this?" No – we are thinking here only about "What is <u>important</u> to me?"

Incidentally, if for some reason you don't make that initial goal, the other 'What?' question to ask is "What did I learn from this?" (rather than "Why did I mess up?", or similar). I first introduced this thought in **GOOAAAALLLLL!!!!!** (page 26).

I have also noticed that, for many people "What did you learn?" initially seems like a funny question to be asked (funny 'peculiar' not funny 'ha ha'), and almost always takes some time to elicit a clear answer. If you wait however, and allow yourself time to process, (to think about your thinking), surprising things can come to the surface! For more thinking on this, check out my **Thought Piece – Get SMART Look Yourself in the i** (page 51).

The bottom line is that, if you clarify the 'What is important?' part, and the 'What did you learn part?' everything else follows, step by step, with each step informing the next.

*As the images unwind, Like the circles that you find,
in the windmills of your mind.*

**Unwind the images – you are outside the circular –
what is important to you?**

thoughts

With a Little Help from Your Friends

On the Beatles legendary 'Sergeant Pepper' Album, Ringo sings …

"I get by with a little help from my friends…"

Leaving aside for the moment the quality of his singing voice (or lack thereof) I am here to tell you that John, Paul, George and Ringo may have hit on something with that sentiment. It appears that 'The Fab Four' were way ahead of the times with their philosophy regarding the relationship between friendship, health and even longevity! The reason I make this bold statement (and an even bolder attempt at singing a few bars of this song while waiting in line at Starbucks) was because I spotted something in the newspaper I picked up there that caught my attention.

An article in *Science Times* (of *The New York Times*) reported on the rapidly increasing amount of research into the importance of friendships and social networks to overall health. Here's the lead paragraph in full

> In the quest for better health, many people turn to doctors,
> self-help books or herbal supplements. But they overlook a
> powerful weapon that could help them fight illness and
> depression, speed recovery, slow aging and prolong life:
> their friends.

The article cited an Australian study which reported that older people with a large circle of friends were '… 22 percent less likely to die' during the study period than those with fewer friends. Also a large US study that reported ' … an increase of almost 60% in the risk of obesity among people whose friends had gained weight'. A recent article in the *American Journal of Public Health*, reported that a Harvard research team followed 16,000 men and women over age 50 for six years. The results showed a clear connection between being socially active and involved, while preserving memory and cognitive abilities. There is increasing evidence to suggest that friendship has an even greater effect on health than a spouse or family member!

This is all highly interesting and valuable information, and more research of course will bring even greater clarity to these connections. In the meantime, however, I want to comment on the way this kind of research is conducted and the way it is reported. In my ongoing quest of pursuing an 'asset-based' approach to health and wellness (See **Kicking Yourself Up the Assets,** page 20), I continually find that 'benefits' are almost always reported as 'reductions in risk' (See **Getting Less Bad,** page 23)

Take the results of the Australian study reported above. The other way of viewing these results is that older people with larger circles of friends were (some percentage) <u>more likely to live</u> – so enabling them to continue to enjoy life. Now, which would you prefer to experience – being less likely to die – or being more likely to live? Of course it's all in the way you (choose to) think about it. However, for me, positive is always preferable to negative. I'd rather 'get more good' than 'get less bad'. I view the US study in the same way. What about the group who had friends that were of normal weight? What positive things happened to them? What is the message being sent when research results are reported in this way? Avoid your friends, or avoid making friends if they are overweight? The point I am trying to make here is that there are many benefits to be gained from building and keeping friendships, perhaps more than we ever realized. More importantly, these benefits are <u>positive</u> experiences, best 'received' (and perhaps even reciprocated!) when expressed in a positive fashion. While the research on friendship is still embryonic, there is a large, and still growing body of research in 'Positive Psychology' that confirms the relationship between positivity and health. Google it when you get a chance

***What is coming up for you as you think about
choosing to be 'positively well'?***

thoughts

Asking the Expert – Making Your Own Difference

When we want to 'make a difference' in our lives (get more active, get fit, be leaner, be more relaxed etc), we often go to an 'expert' for advice, guidance and motivation. After all, an expert is someone who is highly trained and highly knowledgeable. This means that they know what to do. More importantly they know what YOU should do, what you ought to do (and of course what you have been <u>meaning to do</u> for some time!). When you meet with your expert what happens typically follows a common path – a 3 Step approach that I call 'Show and Tell'.

> **Step 1.** You meet with, and talk to an 'expert' about what your goal is (*I want to lose weight, get fit, reduce stress,* etc)

> **Step 2.** After a conversation that varies in length from person to person, the expert first **shows** you what to do *Here's how you work this machine, lift this dumbbell, write out your meal plan, plan your program,* etc, and then **tells** you how to do it, *Follow these steps... directions... advice,* or *Make sure you do it like this... and then this... and then this...*

> **Step 3.** The expert keeps **showing** you and **telling** you in different ways until you do it 'properly'. If you do not succeed in making your goal, the typical expert response is something like

> > *Ok, why do you think you didn't make it?* or maybe
> > *Ok let's try (something different) this time*

By the way, the other thing to mention here is that if you don't 'make it', the fault is almost always assumed to be <u>yours</u> (both by you and by the expert). Maybe you just didn't try hard enough, didn't have the will power, didn't have the commitment etc. Sound familiar?

The rather obvious issue with this approach is that Show and Tell is designed for – and only works in – Kindergarten! My children loved these sessions back then, but have long since outgrown them and moved on to more appropriate discovery methods. However, in my field of exercise, wellness and physical activity, Show and Tell still reigns supreme. The kind of three-step approach I describe above is based on the assumption that if you simply provide intelligent people with important and understandable information about the benefits of healthy behaviors (or, more frequently, the risks of unhealthy behaviors) then they will take this to heart and 'just do it' (with apologies to Nike!). Here's the thing with all this. There really is no question that, assuming the information and instruction provided is accurate, <u>this really would be a highly effective approach for everyone</u>

if only they would do it!

History has shown us, however, that even with the almost limitless availability of health and wellness information in the media and on the web, more people are overweight and sedentary than ever before. It is clear that knowing what to do, or having an expert Show and Tell us what to do, just does not work – but we continue to think this way and act this way regardless!

This is not the fault of the expert, who has often been through rigorous, highly demanding academic training, preparing them for one thing: to offer their own thinking and expertise to the client as to what they should do, and what they need to do. It's also not the fault of the client – who is prepared to believe that the expert knows best – after all that's why they <u>are</u> an expert! The tendency, therefore, is that

- The expert will think (and are trained to think) they know best for the client, and
- The client will think (and are conditioned to think) that the expert knows best for them. That is, after all, why they hired him/her in the first place! No-one is 'at fault' here – it is fault neutral!

*It is time for a new way of thinking –
of making* **Thought Moves**

You can make <u>your own difference</u>! You are a singular and unique individual on this planet, you have your own goals and aspirations, your own motivations and inspirations, your own wants and your own needs your own angels and your own demons. Here's a **Thought** that will **Move** you taken from the Intrinsic Coaching Methodology

– YOU are the expert on you –

No-one knows you better than you – no-one! You know instinctively that this is true, so think about what logically follows. If you pass over responsibility for yourself to someone else – to someone who knows only what they see of you, maybe has only just met you for the first time – to someone who can only work with what you show them – or what is merely apparent to them – how can you realistically expect something important and lasting to happen for you?

If you ask someone to 'prescribe a program' for you – and you take responsibility for doing the program. What you are actually doing is taking responsibility for THAT person's program – for someone else's stuff! After all they made it up FOR YOU. If and when you start, or – like so many others before, re-start such a program – you do so more in hope than expectation. This is no way to achieve a goal. Experts know all about 'cause and effect' – this is their training, this is their knowledge. They know that 'If you do 'this', then 'this' will happen'. However they don't know YOU – they haven't been educated in YOU – they don't have a degree in YOU.

We hear a lot these days about 'personal responsibility' – for health, for being active etc, and we hear about how it's all down to us. At base, this is true of course – responsibility for our health is, in the main, ours. Taking responsibility is a good and desirable thing. However, if you do take responsibility, make sure it's responsibility for something that's yours – not someone else's idea of what is good for you or what you should or shouldn't do. While there is nothing unsafe or dangerous about, e.g. Show and Tell, there is a better way.

"What is important to me? What do I value?"

These are the foundational questions of what *Thought Moves*

What's coming up for you?

thoughts

Thinking INSIDE the Box

The following section contains practical examples of how the **Thought Moves** process can deepen the impact of a well-accepted traditional approach to goal-setting.

Get S.M.A.R.T.!
(Look Yourself in the i)

I don't know how many of you remember the 'Get Smart' TV series of the late '60's – but this **Thought Piece** has nothing at all to do with that show – or the secret agent of the same name who always seemed to be looking for a secret formula stolen by KAOS! Instead this is about a secret modification to another identically named formula for setting goals (Formula S.M.A.R.T.). I am now about to reveal this modification to you…. stand by while I call in to CONTROL on my shoe phone, descend in the super-secret phone booth elevator, untwirl the combination of this safe and de-activate the alarms.

Seriously though…. there really is an acronym S.M.A.R.T. for goal setting and although it is very well known in business, academic and scientific fields (Google-ing 'SMART Goals' gets you more than 631,000,000 hits), I have not seen it often used by 'regular people' (e.g. for those annually ubiquitous New Year's Resolutions).

So what are SMART goals? The whole smart thing came out of an extensive body of research on goal setting which suggested that any goal is more likely to be achieved if you think about it and plan for it in a particular and methodical fashion. The results of this research was boiled down to the finding that a goal is more likely to be achieved if it is 'SPECIFIC', 'MEASURABLE', 'ACHIEVABLE', 'REALISTIC', and 'TIMELY'. If you take the first letter of each of these words it spells SMART – pretty smart eh? I wonder how long it took them to come up with that?

I have taught and applied this process many times, with some success, during my tenure as a university professor. What I have also discovered as an Intrinsic Coach® is that a small modification to this acronym, when acted upon, can make it far more meaningful to the person doing the goal setting. I call this modification iS.M.A.R.T.

The 'i' stands for intrinsically (my favorite), but can also stand for important (my favorite) or inside (my favorite), or increasingly (my favorite), or even I'm (my favorite). The point is that, apart from the fact I have a lot of favorites, more meaningful goal setting comes from that 'i' and is all about what is important to you and only you.

Before you embark on the iS.M.A.R.T. process of setting the goal therefore, it will be essential to first clarify what is important to you (and only to you) about that goal. Ask yourself the two 'Whats'

> *What is my goal? What is important to me about this goal?*

By the way these Whats are asking entirely different questions, although very often they will be thought of as asking the same thing. Here's a common example

> **What is my goal?**
> *Answer:* I want to lose weight
>
> **What is important to me about this goal?**
> *Answer:* I want to lose weight (Duh!)

The second of these questions (What is important to me ...?) is the defining issue here, and, I believe, is the key to all meaningful goal setting and goal achievement. If you can ask and answer this question honestly, (e.g. "What is important to me about losing weight?") you allow your intrinsic values, i.e. what you really want, to be called to awareness from where they are swirling around in your undermind. When you elicit this kind of clarity you will be surprised at what was there all the time, just waiting to be discovered!

> *clarity is in the **i** of the beholder*

Whatever comes up for you, will be more meaningful to you (and only you) in your very own, singular, one of a kind, unique life. Thinking iSMART is thinking intrinsically.

> *So, as you clarify your goal, look yourself in the i –*
> *what are you seeing there? What Thought Moves you?*

thoughts

Thinking iS.M.A.R.T., Specifically

In my last **Thought Piece** I talked about the importance of 'iS.M.A.R.T.' goal setting. Once you have clarified your goal in this way (to see the goal in your minds 'i') the SMART process just clicks in (Specific, Measurable, Achievable, Realistic, Timely).

Although there is a wealth of information out there on SMART goals, I want to offer a different and new way of thinking about this (iThink?) one acronymic letter at a time. Let's start with the 'S' word.

SPECIFIC

Research tells us that if you are specific about the goal you set, you have a much better chance of achieving it. For example "I'm going to walk briskly around the neighborhood for 15 minutes every day" is very specific, whereas 'I'm getting in gear for the rest of the year' or 'I'm going to be lean in 2018" are non-specific, 'fuzzy' goals (even though the rhyming thing may allow the goal to roll off the tongue a little easier!).

So what makes a goal 'specific?

Well, there are lots of suggestions out there (Google them and see!) for making sure that goals are specific, many of which are based on the famous 5 'W's.

Who? What? When? Where? Why?

This is certainly one way to point you in the direction of specificity

Who:	Who else is involved?
What:	What do I want to accomplish?
Where:	Where am I going to do it?
When:	When am I going to do it – and for how long?
Why:	Why am I doing it?

My **Thought Moves** approach here – my 'aha' moment! – is that If you adopt the 'i' approach, these Ws all become assimilated into the two primary, intrinsic 'Whats' I wrote about in **Look Yourself in The i** (page 51).

What do I want?

What is important to me?

Once these two primary 'Whats' have been answered the other Ws just fall into place!

When you answer these two 'Whats' honestly (i.e. intrinsically) everything gets clarified. Once this happens, you have optimized your potential for achieving your goal.

> **So ... specifically... what do you want...**
> **what is important to you about this?**

thoughts

Thinking iS.M.A.R.T., Measurably

The second acronymic letter after the 'i' is

MEASURABLE

Research tells us that a 'Measurable' goal is a 'makeable' goal. I'm summarizing here of course because it is highly unlikely that researchers would be this simplistic. In research terms you would be more likely to read that setting measurable goals allows you to...

> *"Establish concrete criteria for accurately determining progress toward the attainment of each set goal considered to be appropriate for the individual in question"*

But hopefully 'makeable' does it for you.

My point here is that if you can measure the goal you can make the goal. Of course 'Makeable' is no guarantee you <u>are</u> going to make it – just that you are far more likely to do so if you are able to measure what you want to make.

Measurement provides some direction to your goal and puts your achievement into perspective (Did I make it or not? Was I successful or not?). Only by measuring (and being able to measure) will you discover the answers to these indispensable goal-oriented questions.

> *What is your start point? What is your endpoint? How will you know where you end up if you don't know where you started?*

I made the point in my last **Thought Piece** that, with this approach, being Specific in your goal setting was important. Being Measurable is all of a part with this because the more specific your goal is – the easier it is to measure. For example "I'm going to get more active this year" is not specific and not really measurable. How do you know when you have 'got' more active? In contrast, "I'm going to walk briskly around the neighborhood for 15 minutes every day' is not only Specific but also Measurable.

Like this...

Did I walk every day around the neighborhood? Answer = Yes/No.
Did I walk briskly? Answer = Yes/No
Did I walk for 15 minutes? Answer = Yes/No

You see how all these things are coming together?

So ask yourself ...
What measure will tell me I have achieved my goal?

thoughts

Thinking iS.M.A.R.T., Attainably

This seems like the most obvious of the iS.M.A.R.T. letters so far

ATTAINABLY

You mean that if I set a goal it has to be one that I can actually do? – DUH!

On second thinking however this is a factor that deserves closer attention since very often, like beauty, attainment is in the eye (and more importantly the 'i') of the beholder, reminding me of what Henry Ford once famously said

> *'Whether you think you can or you think you can't, you are right'*

Research, and (eventually for some people) experience tells us that the 'best' kind of goals are those that are 'challenging but achievable' – what industry and the corporate world describe as 'stretch' goals, and pop psychologists or self help gurus often describe using motivational rhyming phrases

> *"If you can believe it, you can achieve it" … "if you can sustain it,*
> *you can attain it"… "if you can see it, you can be it" …*
> *"if the glove don't fit you must acquit"*

Well ok, maybe not the last one – but you get what I mean, right?

These phrases and others like them support the idea of something very simplistic like "You can achieve anything you set your mind to" – another popular declaration much loved by parents and anyone that wants their child to be President of the United States. When hearing this statement, even the most positive asset-based person (like me!) is likely to reply… "Anything????' You can achieve <u>anything</u> you set your mind to?' I'd like some clarity on that!"

As I think about Attainment and these kind of phrases, what comes up for me very powerfully is the importance of the 'i' part of iSMART – something I wrote about in the very first thought piece of this series. Seeing things in your mind's 'i' brings up 2 essential, but often underestimated ways of thinking about goal setting and goal attainment

Clarity: *What does this goal look like to you?*
Importance: *What is important to you about this goal?*

So for example ...

You want to lose weight? Ok, what does losing weight look like to you? What is important to you about losing weight?

You want to be more active? Ok, what does being more active look like to you? What is important to you about being more active?

You want to reduce the stress in your life? Ok, what does a stress-free life look like to you? What is important to you about being stress-free?

You want to ... etc

"Any goal you set your mind to", now becomes "Any goal you set *with these two questions in your mind*" (i.e. in your mind's 'i'). These kinds of **Thought Moves** bring up a whole new world of attainment possibilities – with an important qualifier – that turns out to be the next acronymic letter!

So, as you think about this information...

What does attaining this goal look like to you?
What is important to you about attaining this goal?

thoughts

62

Thinking iS.M.A.R.T., Relevantly (Really Importantly)

Ok you probably noticed I added a couple of words here (with tongue ever so slightly in cheek)

RELEVANTLY, REALLY IMPORTANTLY

... and here's why. The 'R' in this acronym is typically written as 'Realistic'. However the issue here (for me anyway) is that this word is hardly any different from our previous word 'Attainable'. After all if something is 'Attainable' it must, by definition, also be 'Realistic'. Apart from these overlapping meanings 'Realistic' is also, in my opinion, the 'shakiest' of the SMART acronym. Here are some goal oriented meanings of 'Realistic' I found recently.

> The goal must be an objective you are 'willing and able to work towards' – It must be 'sensible' – It must be 'wisely planned'.

These are all true of course, though are so obviously self-evident and generic that it is hard to believe they could be of much help to the person seeking to set the goal.

'Relevant' on the other hand has a different context – it has connotations with 'importance' – which brings us back to my earlier **Look Yourself in the i** (page 51) **Thought Piece**.

So I'm going to part with tradition here and say that this 'R' best represents 'Relevant' – in other words something that has meaning for you, and is important for you at the time of setting the goal. It has the added advantage of being able to be defined in terms of your own, unique and current situation, which brings us back to **Look Yourself in the i** (page 51).

So, as you think about this, ask yourself ...

What is relevant to me about achieving this goal?

thoughts

Thinking iS.M.A.R.T., Timely

Effective goal setting is achieved by utilizing the last acronymic letter

TIMELY

Research has told us that goals are best set and completed within a specific time frame, in other words "How long will you give yourself to achieve this goal?"

While a definable, pre-determined time frame is necessary for effective goal achievement, from an Intrinsic Coaching® perspective there are really **two** time frames

What is important to you RIGHT NOW (Timeframe #1)

When will you commit to achieving that goal? (Timeframe #2)

An Intrinsic Coaching® approach to Time takes the goal setting process to a whole new level of involvement. Anchoring the goal commitment to a time frame allows the coach to ask something much more meaningful and far reaching than just "How's it going so far?" A coaching approach to Time provides a valuable context for learning ...

You didn't make the goal in the time frame? What did you learn? What will you do differently?

You did make the goal in the time frame? What did you learn? What will you do differently?

As you think about this – what did you learn over this time – what will you do differently with your goal setting?

thoughts

Thinking iS.M.A.R.T., Accountably

Ok, I introduced another letter here without warning. This last letter is not typically included in the SMART approach to goal setting but, paradoxically, no goal setting and attainment is complete without it

ACCOUNTABILITY

Accountability is an essential - some would say (including me) indispensable – part of a coaching approach to goal setting. For example by asking, "How do you want to be accountable for the actions you have committed to over this period?" or "How do you want to keep track of your progress?", is all a part of the commitment to and accountability for that goal. In this way the goal setter takes ownership of the goal he/she has set. Any number of options could be appropriate for this – email, phone call, text etc.

Research has shown that when goal setters are able to take ownership of, and be accountable for the goals they set, such goals are far more likely to be achieved. Since ownership is in the 'i' of the beholder, the important thing here is that whatever the goal setter commits to will continue to elicit the all important 'i' response.

So, ask yourself... How will I be accountable –
how will I take responsibility for my goal setting?

thoughts

A real-life **Thought Moves** workshop

Thinking About Choices

Reflective Pondering

When you think about setting goals, you are really thinking about deciding something. You are, essentially, <u>choosing</u> a path or an action that is important to you – what you are wanting – what you value.

However these values are often buried under deep layers of conventional, and almost reflexive 'Should' and 'Ought' thinking. "What should I do?" ... "I ought to do this" etc.

One way of clarifying your Choices – your 'wants' vs your 'wannabes', your 'values' vs your 'vanities' is to immerse yourself in what I call 'Reflective Pondering' – where your **Thought Moves** are involved in an inwardly spiraling process.

An example of how this process can work appears on the next few pages. I have based it on my past experiences of actual answers from real persons

By the way this experiment does not have to be completed in a single session – and is probably more effective if your answers are allowed to emerge over time – without any forcing or concentrated thinking.

Here's how it works...

First, choose your goal. Something that you have been wanting for yourself. Something that is important to you. Something that you may even have tried before. It can be something you want now, or something you want for the future. There are no limitations: it only has to be something that makes sense to you at the time.

Once you have done this... move on to the following pages.

Thinking About Choices

Reflective Pondering Example

Note: This is based on a real life conversation with a client.

Let's say your goal is...
'By the end of 12 weeks I will walk 5 miles at a brisk pace without stopping'

> **Step 1.** Ask yourself "<u>What is important to me</u>...?" about this goal.
> *What is important to me about walking 5 miles at a brisk pace without stopping?*
> **THEN:** Think about (reflect on) this question, and write down your answer in this format
> For example...
> *If I was able to walk 5 miles at a brisk pace without stopping... I would be fitter*

> **Step 2.** Ask, '<u>What is important to me</u>...?' about this new answer
> *What is important to me about being fitter?*
> **THEN:** Think about (reflect on) this new question, and write down your answer as before
> For example...
> *If I was fitter ... I would feel good about myself and what I had achieved*

> **Step 3.** Ask, '<u>What is important to me</u>...?' about this new answer
> *What is important to me about feeling good about myself and what I had achieved?*
> **THEN:** Think about (reflect on) this question, and write down your answer as before
> For example...
> *If I felt good about myself and what I had achieved ... I would be more likely to take on bigger challenges*

> **Step 4.** Ask, '<u>What is important to me</u>...?' about this new answer
> *What is important to me about taking on bigger challenges?*
> **THEN:** Think about (reflect on) this question, and write down your answer as before

For example...
If I was able to take on bigger challenges ... I would get out more and meet people

Step 5. Ask, 'What is important to me...?' about this new answer
What is important to me about getting out more and meeting new people?
THEN: Think about (reflect on) this question, and write down your answer as before
For example...
If I got out more and met new people... I would be more confident in company

Step 6. Ask, 'What is important to me...?' about this new answer
What is important to me about being more confident in company?
THEN: Think about (reflect on) this question, and write down your answer as before
For example...
If I was more confident in company ... etc.

You see how the 'importance' – and so the valuing – shifts to a deeper level? It started off with a goal of being 'fitter', something external/extrinsic to the person, that, for most individuals, would be an end in itself. However, it ended up with something much deeper and internal/intrinsic to the person.

Even though this is only one reality-based example, I have witnessed many occasions where reflective pondering (***Thought Moves***) like this has worked in much the same way. Deeper thinking and deeper values can come to light if they are allowed space and time to 'germinate' through this kind of thinking. You may be surprised what you discover is important to you by the end of your very own 'inwardly spiraling' process! BTW, there is no set number of Steps. See where you are at Step 10.

Take a sheet of paper and try this for yourself
See what comes up for you – Step by self-reflective Step!

What emerges from your *Thought Moves*
is all about what is important to YOU –
what you VALUE

thoughts

Next Steps

The Thinking Behind Choices

A brief introduction to Valuing
– Its measurement and application –

The Hartman/Marshall Synthesis

While the workshop example above was focused on the value of Thinking <u>about</u> Choices, the final phase of this book is focused on the Thinking <u>behind</u> Choices. Something that takes valuing to a whole new level!

Choices

Every action we take in life is the result of a choice of some kind, whether conscious or unconscious. But what is it that underpins – or undermines – a person's capacity to take action to change something in their life? Something that they say they want to change – but often also say they have repeatedly tried and 'failed' to change. In other words, that what they <u>chose to do</u> was unsuccessful – although they rarely think about it in those terms.

Thought Moves, up to this point, has addressed a very basic approach to this kind of 'Change Thinking'. However, there are deeper, more 'choiceful' ways of making decisions. The final section of this book introduces what I believe is the most powerful of these.

The Thinking Behind Choices

Whatever change we desire, we typically approach it head on with a 'What can I do?' kind of thinking. We set about working out what to do, in a sensible, logical, rational kind of way. We may think of alternative choices, make a plan, or make a pros and cons list. However, this approach rarely works, and the reason – almost always – is because of <u>the way we think</u> about what we want to change.

Here's the thing. When you are making relatively straightforward choices such as where to spend your holidays, what car to buy, what color to paint the family room, what brand of toothpaste to use, etc., your deliberate, logical, 'pros and cons' approach may work well. However, when you are wrestling with more complex lifestyle issues such as relationships, career decisions, weight loss, body image, becoming more active etc., your best thinking will emerge from a more patient, intrinsic, pondering approach. A kind of thinking that is concerned not with the <u>content</u> of your thinking (Thinking about **What** you think), but with the <u>process</u> of your thinking (Thinking about **How** you think).

This thinking about thinking, something that I call "meta-thinking", often transpires in your deepest thoughts, those below the level of your consciousness: thoughts that emerge only when they are allowed time to 'germinate'. This is where your values reside – and your values are at the heart of your innermost feelings, your deepest held beliefs. Your best thinking – and so your best choices <u>for you</u> – originate from your values.

This kind of thinking is a skill that can be learned, and if we are 'true to ourselves' in this way, we will experience a clarity of thought that will lead to better decision making.

> *The actions we take emerge from the choices we make, the choices we make emerge from the thinking behind those choices. Being aware of this thinking allows our values to come to awareness and leads to better choices.*

Values and Self Knowledge – A Brief Introduction

The unique importance of values, and a formal way of measuring valuing and valuation, was first proposed by Dr. Robert Hartman, a German scientist and philosopher who in the mid-1900s, developed the theory and practice of Axiology - the science of value. He also developed the specialized mathematics of value on which Axiology is based, and was nominated for the Nobel Peace Prize in 1973 because of his work in this area.

> *Our values are the keys to our personalities, to self-knowledge, and to understanding others.*
> ~ Dr. Robert S Hartman

Based on this work, Dr. Hartman developed a unique values profiling and measurement questionnaire now known universally as The Hartman Value Profile (HVP). It is one of the most powerful and highly regarded profiling systems in the world, and the only one founded in Mathematics. Its more recent application as a powerful coaching tool emerged from the visionary work of Christina Marshall, Founder of Intrinsic Solutions International, who synthesized her thinking with the work of Dr. Hartman.

The Hartman/Marshall Synthesis process begins with an online questionnaire that produces a comprehensive HVP Report. This in itself provides uniquely personalized information about the choices and behaviors of the participant.

However, the real power behind this approach is in the conversation that develops from discussing the report one-on-one with a Certified Valuation Specialist (CVS). It is from here that true clarity about lifestyle choices emerges and continues to emerge over time.

> *It isn't knowledge about thinking that is lacking. It isn't a lack of things to think about that is the main problem. It is awareness-in-progress of our processes of thinking, and making awareness of those processes more important than awareness of the content of our thinking.*
> ~ Christina Marshall

The HVP is an online questionnaire provided by a European profiling company 'profiling**values**' (www.profilingvalues.com) who are collaborating partners with Christina Marshal and Intrinsic Solutions International.

Each individual who completes the questionnaire will receive a unique Profile Report that reflects the capacities and values that make sense to them at that time. The Profile and the coach/coachee conversation resulting from it is used as a vehicle for clarifying the *Thinking Behind Choices* that individuals make, and are making in their lives. In other words – how **Thought Moves** them.

> **As Dr. Seuss says (in a different context) –**
> **"Oh the places you'll go!"**

A Special Offer for YOU!

If you want to experience the life changing power of
The Hartman/Marshall Synthesis and
the Thinking Behind Choices ...

Take the Next Step!

Accept a free, no-obligation, 15-minute consultation
and begin to discover how **Thought Moves** you.

Contact Me

(602) 793-0752

**wphillips@thoughtmoves.com
www.thoughtmoves.com**

thoughts

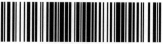

Made in the USA
Columbia, SC
19 December 2018